Homemade Hair Care:

34 Natural Toxic-Free Recipes with Essential Oils for Your Hair

Table of content:

Introduction: You're tired of the chemicals.

You've tried just about every hair product out there to make your hair look and feel healthy. The problem is the more you paid, the more chemicals were in the products and the more you had to purchase to cleanse your hair of the residue. You started looking online for a natural alternative, but your head spun with all the recipes, advice, and ingredients, not knowing which was actually good for your hair and which ones you needed to avoid. This book will provide, not only the answers you're looking for, but the breakdown of all the ingredients and recipes to start making your own at home. From what you need to how to make it, we will give you all you need to take charge of your own scalp and hair health.

Chapter 1 - Your Scalp and Hair

You scratch it when it itches. You scratch it when you brush it, and you pull it when you style your hair. It's your scalp, and it needs as much attention as your hair. If you scalp is dry or unhealthy, it reflects in your hair, making it either dull and dry, or oily.

Dandruff

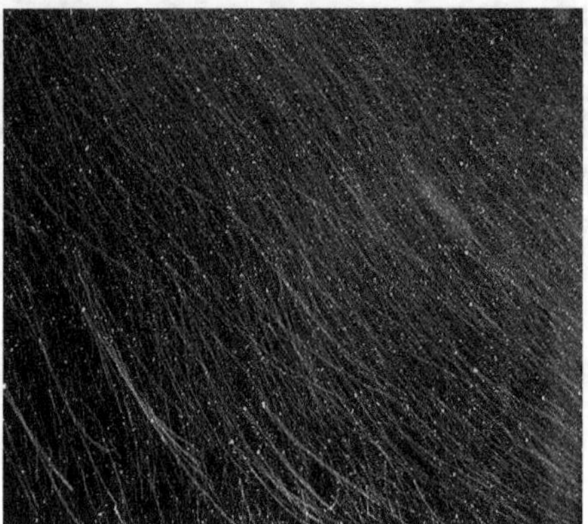

This is the flaking of your scalp when its too dry to retain the natural sebum the sabaceous glands produce. These flakes can be small, only being seen when you scratch your scalp, or large enough to be noticed by anyone who looks.

How your hair gets damaged

Your hair takes a ton of abuse. With every curling or straightening iron and blow drying session, your hair can sustain damage. You can dry out your hair when you wash it too often, over style it, and even bleach and dye your hair. Doing any of these things can leave your hair dry, stringy, brittle, and very susceptible to breaking and split ends.

When you shampoo and condition your hair, it's clean, a little too clean in some instances, making your scalp work overtime to make the sebum, or natural oil, to keep itself moisturized. This can lead to hair looking oily just 24 hours after you have washed it. There is a way to reset the balance to your scalp. It's called the:

No Shampoo Method

You only need the following ingredients to get started:
Baking soda
Water
Unfiltered Apple Cider Vinegar
Empty shampoo bottle
Two-cup measuring cup

• In a standard size bottle of water, add two tsp of baking soda and shake until it mixes into the water.

• Put a little on your palm. If it's a little slippery, than it's perfect. If not, add a little more into the water.

• In your measuring cup, add two tablespoons of apple cider vinegar.

• Fill the rest with water.

In the shower:

• Wet your hair
• Work with baking soda solution into your hair.
• Use the vinegar solution to rinse and leave it in. This will restore the pH or your scalp.

Essential Oil

It will take up to seven weeks for your hair to reset, using the technique above once a week until you don't need to use it any longer. You can add essential oils to the vinegar. Here are a couple than can help balance the scalp:

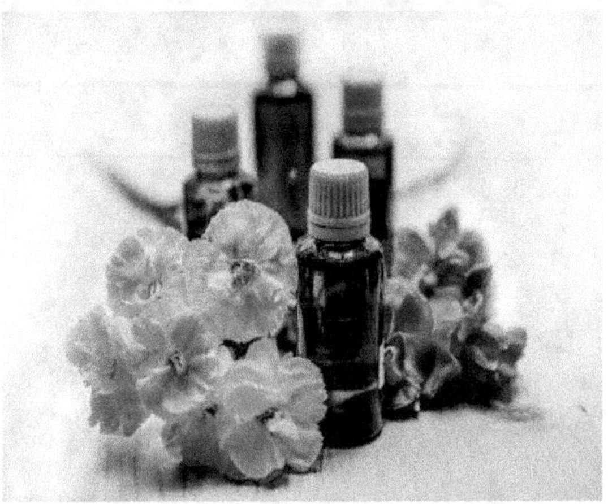

Carrot Seed (Daucus carota)

This is also known as wild carrot. It helps to revitalize the scalp.

Cedarwood (Cedrus atlantica)

This is an essential oil that can help treat dandruff and also promote hair growth. Do not use this oil if pregnant.

Chamomile, Roman (Chamaemelum nobile)

This is a great essential oil for all skin conditions form head to toe. It helps promote healthy hair and scalp.

Clary Sage (Salvia sclarea)

This essential oil is often used to help thinning hair, promote a healthy scalp, fight dandruff, and control oils produced from the sabaceous gland. Do not use if pregnant. It doesn't mix when if you use before you drink alcohol.

Cypress (Cupressus sempervirens)
This oil is used to balance the skin and scalp. It helps to reduce sebum from overactive glands, and regulates the sebum production.

Helichrysum (Helichrysum angustifolium)

This will help with extremely dry scalp.

Lavender (Lavandula angustifolia)

This is an all-purpose essential oil that is good for a skin types. It is often added to shampoos and rinses for dandruff.

Lemon (Citrus limon)

This helps to regulate oily skin and scalp. This can speed a sun burn if used right before going outside.

Patchouli (Pogostemon cablin)

This oil is used often in aromatherapy for hair care, oily hair and skin, and it is also good in treating dandruff.

Rosemary (Rosmarinus officinalis)

This essential oil comes highly recommended for regulating sebum production, stimulating the scalp, helping with thinning hair, ,promoting hair growth, lice, and dandruff. However, it is to be avoided if you are epileptic or suffer from hypertension.

Tea Tree (Melaleuca alternifolia)

This is good for treating dandruff and lice.

Thyme (Thymus vulgaris)

This is another essential oil that can help treat lice. It is also good for regulating oily skin and scalp. This one is however needs to be avoided in cases of hypertension, and pregnancy.

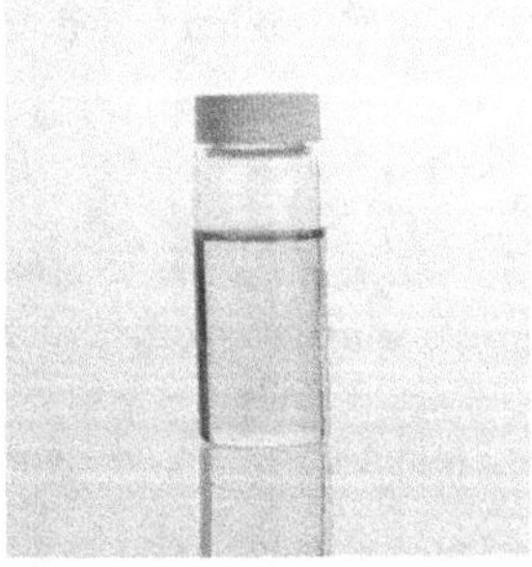

Ylang Ylang (Cananga odorata)

It helps to stimulate hair growth and makes a good ingredient for hair rinses.
As you can see, there are a lot of essential oils you can tailor to your specific needs in terms of hair care. All of the hair care products you tend to buy in the store cannot do that. They are made for a general hair problem and not an individual.

Chapter 2 - Shampoos

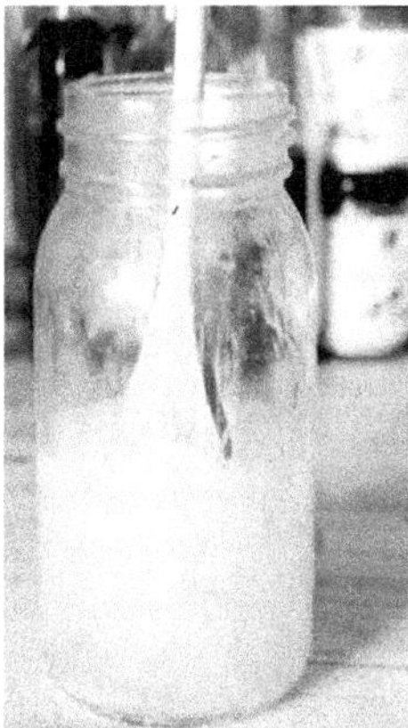

From the most expensive to the ones that only cost a few dollars, all shampoos have chemicals in them that your hair does not need. I will list over a few of these here:

Parabens

These can mimic estrogen, which leads to an imbalance of this hormone in the system and increase the risk of breast cancer. Other names for Parabens are methylparaben, propylparaben, isoparaben, and butylparaben.

Pthalates

This is an ingredient found in items with fragrances that can trigger respiratory problems such as asthma and bronchitis.

1,4-diaxane

This is classified as an animal carcinogen. The FDA, however, allows this compound in shampoos, facial cleansers, and toothpaste. It can also be found in organic products. There are more than 56 ingredients that are related to this compound some of these include:

-sodium laureth sulfate

-sodium myreth sulfate

-polyethylene glycol

-ingredients ending in xynol, ceteareth, and oleth.

Diethanolamine (DEA)

This is an ever-present elmulsifier. Emulsifiers keep the other ingredients in a recipe blended. Up to two-thirds of the products with this chemical in it do not rinse cleanly, leaving DEA to linger on the skin and cause irritation. Cancer, more specifically lung and liver, have been reported, but only if it is a high dose. Other names for this chemical are:

-cocamide DEA

-DEA-cetyl phosphate

-olemide DEA

Formaldehyde

Yes, this is the compound used in preserving human remains and biological specimens. It is often used to smooth hair and skin in soaps and shampoos. It may make you nauseous, cough and can also trigger asthma. They are sneaky with this one, often calling it FRP or some of these names:

-quaternium-15

-dimethyl-dumethyl (DMDM) hydantoin

-imidazolidinyl urea

-sodium hydroxymethylglycinate

Making your own hair care products takes all of these chemicals out of the equation.

You will need a few things to get started making your own shampoo. You probably have these in your kitchen already.

Food Scale

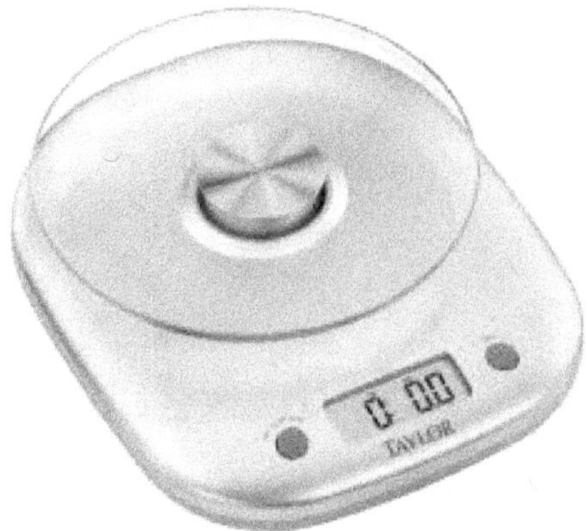

You will be measuring the soap that goes into your shampoo.

Melt and pour soap or Doctor's Bronner's bar soap

You can find melt and pour soap in any craft store, but if you're not comfortable using it, you can purchase Doctor Bronner's Castile Soaps. They do not have the chemicals above.

Empty Shampoo Bottle

You can use any you already have at hand. Just make sure it's rinsed really well.

Blender

This will mix all the ingredients of the shampoo together.

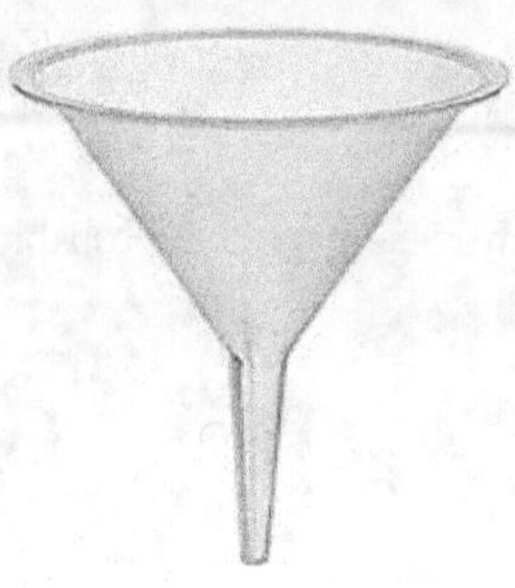

Funnel

This will help you put the shampoo in the bottle of your choice.

Label

This is to label your shampoo and include the ingredients you used to make it.

Oils

Here is a short list of oils commonly used to make homemade shampoo:

Coconut Oil

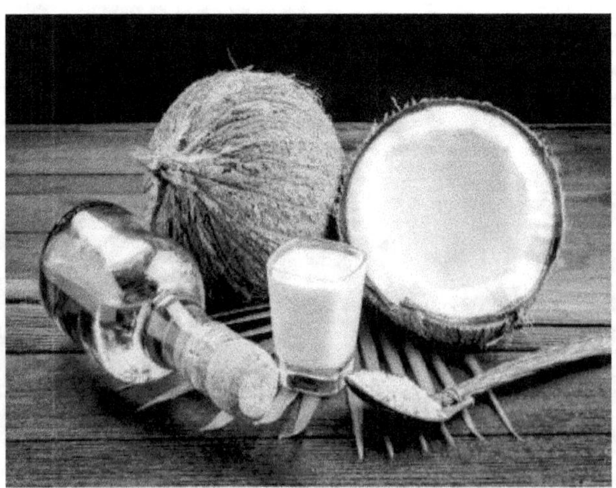

This is rich in minerals and vitamins to nourish your skin. It can also help with frizzing. You will need to get the fractionated version of this oil as the more commonly used version of this oil hardens in temperatures of 76 degrees and below.

Olive oil

This is not the Extra Virgin, but the first press. This oil is darker. Olive oil contains high amounts of vitamin E which is good for the scalp and hair.

Jojoba oil

More a wax than an oil, but it is an oil when in room temperature. This is the closest thing to the sebum your glands produce and can help to bring moisture to hair and a balance to the natural oils in your scalp.

Basic Recipe

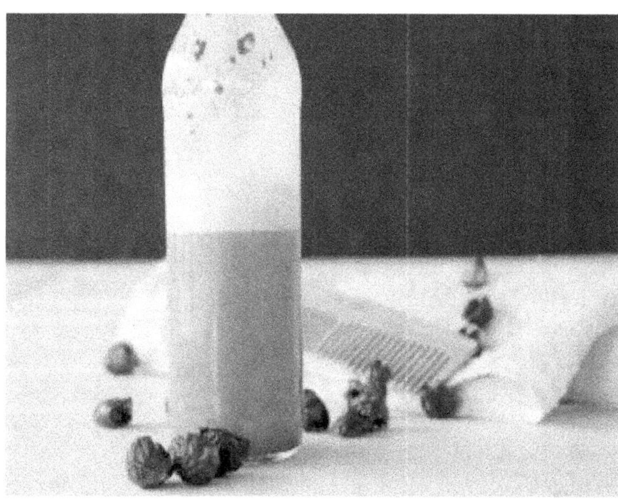

There is a simple recipe for making homemade soap:

4 ounces of Melt and pour or Doctor Bronner's bar soap

1/4 oil

Boiled or filtered water.

50 drops of essential oil

- Grate the soap into a blender.
- Add the oil
- Mix on blend
- Slowly add up to 3/4 cup of water while it is blending.
- Switch to liquify.
- Funnel into the shampoo bottle you are going to use.

If you feel the shampoo is too thick, you can add more water. The shampoo will separate, if you don't use it for a while. This is normal as there are no emulsifiers to keep it from doing so. Because there are no phosphates, it may not lather up as you expect shampoo to do. This is also normal. Your hair is still getting clean, just without extra bubbles.

Dry Scalp I

1/4 Cup Jojoba Oil

10 Drops Carrot Essential Oil

15 Drops Lavender Essential Oil

15 Helichrysum Essential oil

10 Drops Cedarwood Essential Oil

Dry Scalp II

1/4 Cup Coconut Oil

10 Drops Rosemary Essential Oil

15 Drops Cypress Essential Oil

15 Drops Chamomile, Roman Essential Oil

10 Drops Clary sage Essential oil

Dandruff Shampoo

1/4 Cup Olive oil

10 Drops Cedarwood Essential Oil

10 Drops Patchouli Essential Oil

15 Drops Cypress Essential Oil

15 Drops Lavender Essential Oil

Moisturizing Scalp Treatment

2 Eggs (Yes eggs)

10 Drops of Lavender Essential Oil

15 Drops Carrot Essential Oil

15 Drops Helichrysum Essential Oil

- Mix the essential oils, set aside
- Whisk the eggs
- Whisk the essential oils into the eggs.

How to use:

1. Working into damp hair and cover with shower cap.
2. Leave in for twenty minutes
3. Shampoo with dandruff shampoo
4. Use following vinegar rinse.

Vinegar Rinse I

2 Tablespoons Apple Cider Vinegar, unfiltered.

2 Cups water

6 Drops Ylang Ylang Essential Oil

6 Drops Cypress Essential Oil

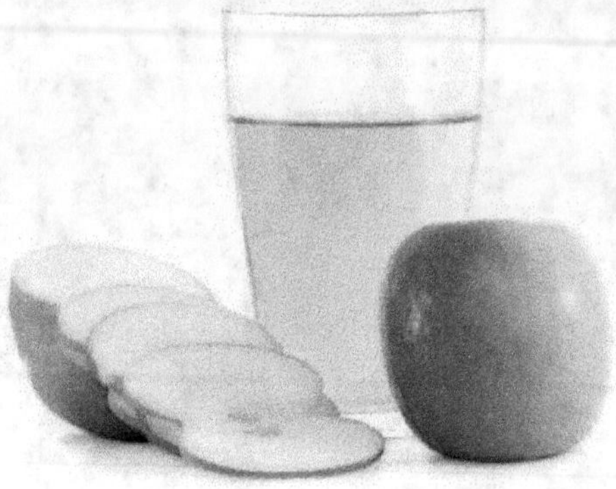

- Mix the essential oils
- Add them to the Apple cider vinegar
- Mix well before adding water. The vinegar not only helps to condition the scalp, but as an emulsifier for the essential oils so they mix better with the water.

How to use:

1. Tilt head backwards in shower or tub.
2. Starting with the front-most hair line, slowly pour the solution so that it soaks into the hair.
3. Use a comb to make sure it evenly distributes on the scalp.
4. Dry and style hair as normal.

Oily Hair

Over washing is one of the many causes of oily scalp and hair. One shouldn't really wash their hair more than three times a week, but most wash daily to get the right style before going to work or out for the evening. Having a naturally oily complexion can normally mean your scalp is oily as well. One has to strike the perfect balance of essential oils in their shampoo and lighter oils in the mix so as not to make it worse.

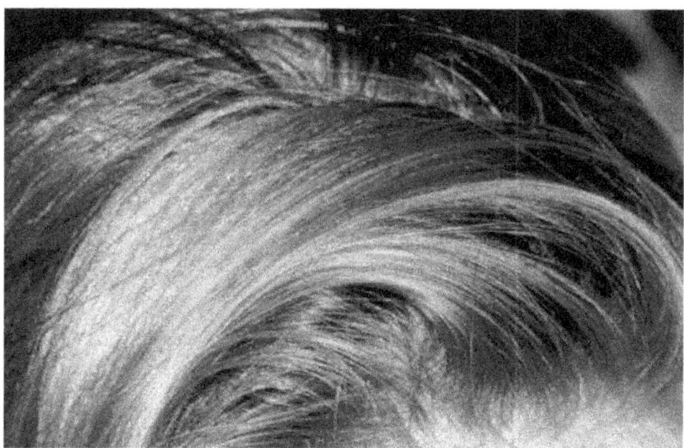

Oils

Sweet Almond Oil

This is a light oil that is packed with the minerals you hair needs without adding to the oily feel of the other oils above.

Apricot Kernel Oil

This has many of the properties of Sweet Almond and thus is a good substitute if you are allergic to tree nuts.

Grapeseed oil

This oil is perhaps the better of the three on this list, but it is a bit more pricey. It provides nutrients to condition the hair and scalp as well as feed it to insure its health.

Essential Oils

There isn't much to add to the list, but there is three more you can add to the mix for helping with excess sebum.

Geranium (Pelargonium graveolens)

This essential oil comes in handy for those with an oily scalp. It helps to curve oils.

Grapefruit (Citrus x paradisi)

This helps to grow the hair. It helps to stem oils created by the skin and scalp.

West Indian Bay (Pimenta racemosa)

This is a scalp stimulant and make a good rinse for dandruff and greasy hair. It also promotes hair growth. Use in small doses and not very often. Since it isn't a more commonly known essential oil, it may be a bit pricey.

Oily Hair I

1/4 Cup Sweet Almond oil
10 Drops Grapefruit Essential Oil
10 Drops Geranium Essential Oil
15 Drops Lavender Essential Oil
15 Drops Cypress Essential Oil

Oily Hair II

1/4 Cup Grapeseed Oil
10 Drops West Indian Bay Essential Oil
10 Drops Thyme Essential Oil
15 Drops Rosemary Essential Oil
15 Drops Carrot Essential Oil

Dry Shampoo

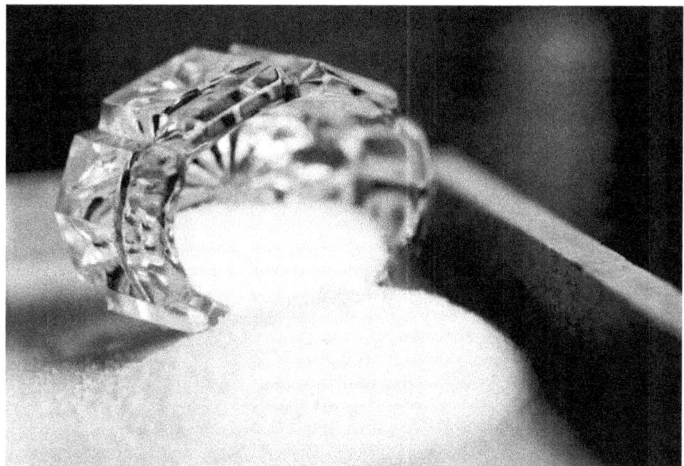

These are "shampoos" that are designed to absorb excess oils in the scalp and used as a stop gap between shampoo sessions:

1. Lightly dab a small amount along part lines.
2. Shake the hair from the root to allow the dry shampoo to fall to the scalp.
3. Take a brush and brush out as much of the hair as possible.

There are one of two things you will need for the dry shampoo:

• Corn starch for light hair
• Cocoa for brown/darker hair.

Dry Shampoo I

1 cup Corn Starch or Cocoa

2 Tablespoons Sweet Almond Oil

6 Drops Lavender Essential Oil

3 Drops Carrot Seed Essential Oil

3 Drops Grapefruit Essential oil

1 cup Corn Starch or Cocoa

2 Tablespoons of Grapeseed

4 Drops Cedarwood Essential Oil

2 West Indian Bay Essential Oil

4 Drops Cypress Essential Oil

- Mix the oils together
- Mix the dry ingredient into the oils.
- Place the shampoo in a tightly lidded container.

Chapter 3 - Conditioner

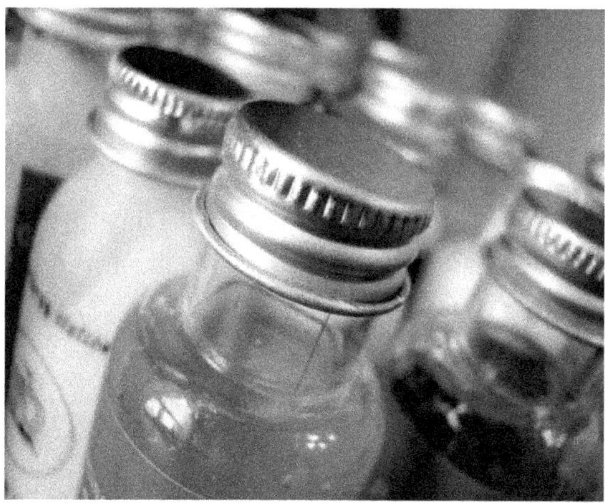

First you shampoo your hair to cleanse it of dirt, sweat, and grit. Then you need to condition it to keep it healthy and strong to prevent breaking. There are typically three types of conditioning:

1. Leave-in
2. Rinse-out
3. Hair mask

The only problem with the second one is that, when you rinse it, you wash most, if not all of it out of your hair, not leaving in enough time to condition the hair or scalp. If it does stay in long enough, it can weigh down the hair.

Leave-in conditioners, sometimes called rinses, are light and designed to stay in the hair, providing extra moisture. This sounds like a good idea, but one good rain and it rinses out, especially if you've done you hair that day.

Hair masks are the type of conditioning masks that stay in for about twenty minutes and then you can wash it out as normal with shampoo.

This are great for infusing your hair with the proteins and minerals you hair needs to get its shine and health back from the abuse everyday styling can do to it. Since these are more intense, by way of conditioning, it isn't recommended you use hair masks no more than once or twice a week, spacing it out by four days.

Moisturizing your hair will help prevent split ends, drying, and breaking. It will also keep your scalp moisturized and healthy, promoting healthy hair as it grows from the shaft. A healthy scalp leads to healthy hair. Here are a few ways you can condition your scalp and hair.

Vinegar Rinse I

2 Cups Water
2 Tablespoons Apple Cider Vinegar unfiltered
6 Drops Ylang Ylang Essential Oil
6 Drops Grapefruit Essential Oil

Vinegar Rinse II

2 Cups Water
2 Tablespoons Apple Cider Vinegar unfiltered
3 Drops Sandalwood Essential Oil
5 Drops Lavender Essential Oil
4 Drops Cypress Essential Oil

Hair Masks

This may sound a bit weird, but hair masks work like facials for your hair and scalp. They nourish your hair, can repair the damage done through styling, and even promote hair growth if your hair is thinning. Hair masks can also provide much needed moisture to your scalp and hair, making it less frizzy and more manageable.

Avocado and Egg Mask (dry scalp)

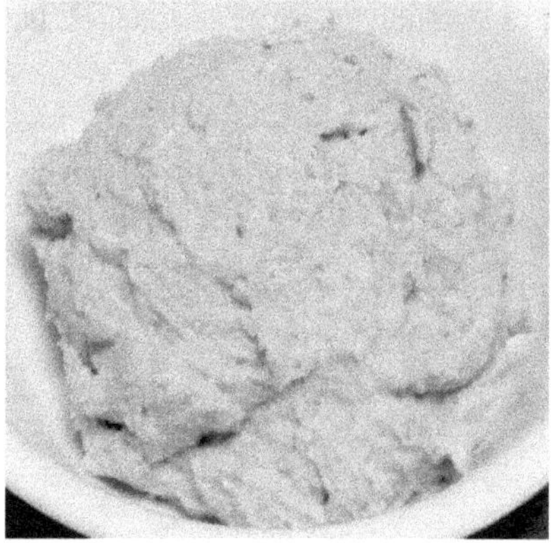

Eggs are an excellent source of protein and avocados provide your hair with oils that can help condition it.

1/2 and Avocado
2 Egg yolks
10 Drops Carrot Essential oil
10 Drops Rosemary Essential oil
20 Drops Lavender Essential oil
10 Drops Sandalwood Essential oil

- Mix the essential oils separately
- Mash the avocado
- Mix the egg yolks into the avocado well
- Mix in the essential oils

How to use:

1. Work into damp hair.
2. Leave in for 15-20 minutes
3. Rinse out in the shower
4. Apply one of the vinegar rinses

Honey and Yogurt Mask (dry scalp)

Honey is sticky and can be a pain to get out of anything once it's been applied, but when you mix with other ingredients, it becomes easy to rinse out.

1 tsp olive oil

1 tsp honey, preferably raw and unfiltered

1/4 Cup yogurt

10 Drops Patchouli Essential oil

10 Drops of Cypress Essential oil

5 Drops of Clary Sage Essential oil

- Mix the essential oil separately from the other ingredients
- Mix the honey and olive oil
- Add the essential oils to the honey and olive oil
- Whisk them into the yogurt

Use as directed for the egg and avocado recipe.

Avocado and Egg (Oily Scalp) I

1/2 and Avocado

2 Egg yolks

10 Drops Lemon Essential oil

10 Drops Cypress Essential oil

15 Drops Ylang Ylang Essential Oil

Directions as above.

Honey Yogurt Mask (Oily Scalp) II

1 tsp olive oil

1 tsp honey, preferably raw and unfiltered

1/4 Cup yogurt

15 Drops Grapefruit Essential oil

5 Drops Rosemary Essential oil

10 Drops Sandalwood Essential oil

5 Drops Carrot Seed Essential oil

Follow Direction as above

Maintenance Mask

This is a simple mask to keep your hair shiny and healthy.

1 tsp olive oil

1 tsp honey, preferably raw and unfiltered

1/4 Cup yogurt

10 Drops Ylang Ylang Essential oil

10 Drops Carrot Seed Essential oil

10 Drops Cypress Essential oil

Follow directions as above.

Chapter 4 - Hair styling products

Now, we're getting to the crux of the matter. It's one thing to make natural products for your hair to condition and clean it, but it is exponentially harder to find all natural products to style and treat your hair. Don't worry. Here are some recipes to get you started.

Mousses and Gels

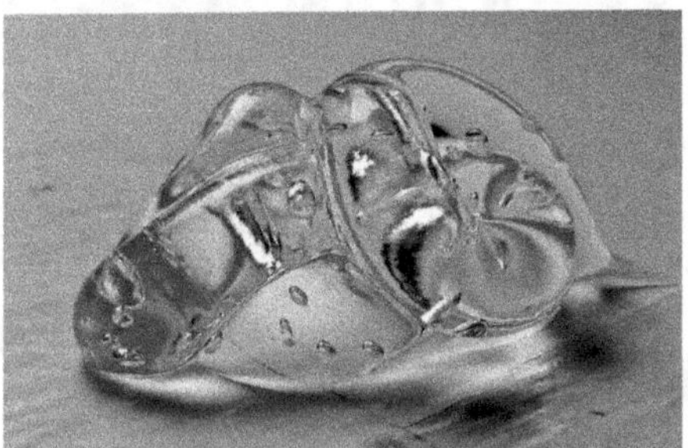

These are the two most popular methods of styling hair. They both help to retain you style, but their difference in consistency means you can't use them for all types of hair.

Mousse

This is typically used for people with naturally curly hair to keep the curls and manage the frizz without compromising the natural bounce of the curls. This also works well for permed curls.

Gels

This product is mostly used for straight hair when trying to maintain a curly style or to keep up a certain look. People with curly hair use it to crunch their curls to make them tight.

Hair Pomade/Balm

This product looks like a cream and is usually sold in either tubes or a container resembling facial cream. It is used to smooth out frizz and make the hair a little more manageable. It doesn't take much to get the results you need. A small pea-sized amount will do the trick. Rub it in your hands and then work it into your hair.

Hair Mousse Basic Recipe

No matter the essential oils you add to your homemade mousse, the basic recipe is the same.

1/2 Cup Shea Butter (moisturizing for the hair)
1/4 Cup Coconut oil (Nutrients for the hair)
1/4 cup Olive oil

• Melt the Shea Butter with the Coconut oil and whip it with a hand mixer for ten minutes
• Add the essential oils while mixing
• Drizzle in the olive oil while mixing
• Add the finished product in a tightly lidded container.

Dry Hair Mousse

10 Drops Carrot Seed Essential oil
20 Drops Lavender Essential oil
20 Drops Cypress Essential oil
20 Drops Roman Chamomile Essential oil
10 Drops Tea Tree Essential oil

Oily Hair Mousse

20 Drops Grapefruit essential oil

10 Drops of Rosemary Essential oil

10 Drops of Ylang Ylang Essential oil

20 Drops of Geranium Essential oil

10 Drops of Sandalwood Essential oil

10 Drops of Lavender Essential oil

Basic Gel Recipe

1/4 tsp pure, unflavored gelatin

1/2 Cup Hot water

- Bring the water to boiling
- Stir in the gelatin.
- When it cools to warm, add your essential oils.

For Dry Hair

10 Drops Cypress Essential oil

10 Drops Lavender Essential oil

5 Drops Helichrysum Essential oil

5 Drops Clary Sage Essential oil

For Oily Hair

10 Drops Grapefruit Essential oil

10 Drops Carrot Seed Essential oil

10 Drops Geranium Essential oil

Hair Pomade/Balm Basic Recipe

1 Ounce Organic Beeswax

1.5 Ounces of Shea Butter

2 Ounces Jojoba Oil

- Melt the beeswax in a double boiler
- Melt in the Shea Butter
- Stir in the Jojoba oil
- As it is cooling, add the essential oils

Dry Hair

10 Drops Patchouli Essential oil

10 Drops Ylang Ylang Essential oil

10 Drops of Roman Chamomile Essential oil

Oily Hair

10 Drops Grapefruit Essential oil

10 Drops Cypress Essential oil

10 Drops Carrot Seed Essential oil

Hair Spray

You've got the mousse, the gel, and the pomade. All you need is the hairspray to keep it all in place. There are two basic recipes you can use, one with sugar and one without.

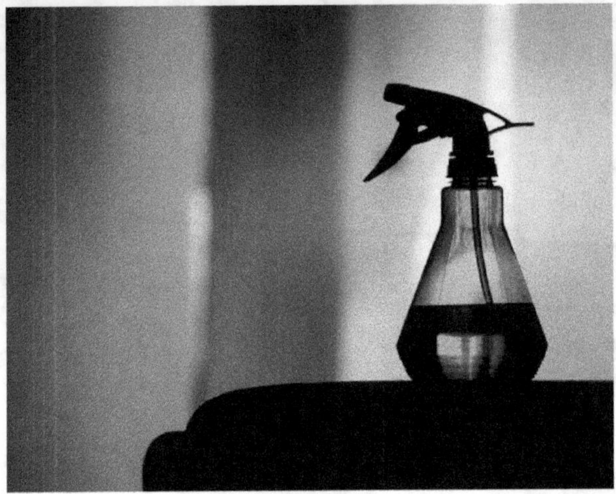

1 Whole Organic Orange (for dark hair) or Organic Lemon (for light hair)

2 Cups distilled or filtered water

2-3 Tbsp High Proof Vodka (or other clear alcohol)

* Wedge the fruit and place it in a pot.
* Add the water and bring to a boil
* Reduce the liquid to half by boiling it down.
* Strain through a cheesecloth to get all of the juice out of the fruit.
* You should have one cup by this time.
* Funnel into a spray bottle after it has cooled.
* Add your essential oils until they are mixed in well.

Sugar Hairspray

1.5 Cups filtered water

2 tablespoons white sugar

1 tablespoon high proof clear alcohol, like vodka

10-15 Drops of essential oils

- Boil water to dissolve the sugar
- Add essential oils to the alcohol
- Add the alcohol solution to the sugar water
- Shake well.
- Adjust the sugar level to increase or decrease the hold of the hairspray.

You can add the following essential oils to the hairspray. The only trick is to wait until the solutions have cooled and shake well.

Luster

20 Drops Ylang Ylang
10 Drops Carrot Seed Essential oil

Moisture

20 Drops Lavender Essential oil
10 Roman Chamomile Essential oil
You can mix and match essential oils to have different aromas for your hairspray.

Chapter 5 - Thinning Hair

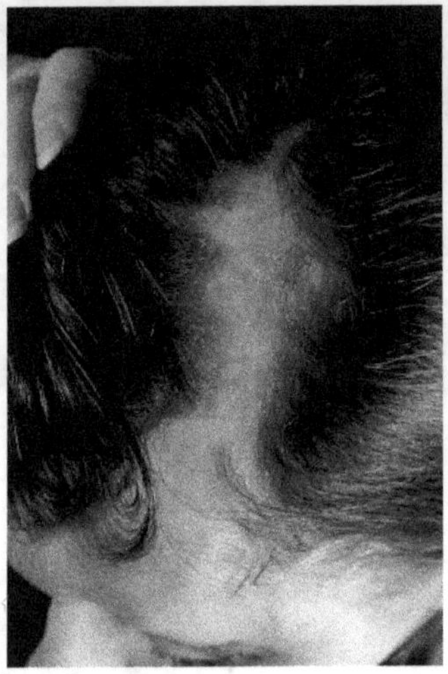

There are several reasons for thinning hair and hair loss. Heredity, stress, and malnutrition are three known causes, but there are some recipes you can make to help keep from losing more, and in some cases, grow some of it back.

The following recipes should be used three times a week.

There really aren't essential oils to add to this list. So I will list the ones from the previous chapter:

Carrot Seed

Cedarwood

Chamomile, Roman

Clary Sage

Lavender

Rosemary

West Indian Bay

This is a basic base to use for the essential oils.

- 4 tsp Jojoba Oil
- 4 tsp Coconut Oil

To Use:

If you are bald:

1. Massage into scalp and let it settle into the scalp
2. Wash with one of the shampoos a previous chapter.
3. Follow up with a vinegar rinse and work it into the scalp.

If you have a thinning spot:

1. Part the hair
2. With your finger tips, work the recipe into the part.
3. Repeat until the thinning spot is worked with the recipe.
4. Place shower cap on your head.
5. Leave in for 15 minutes
6. Wash hair with one of the shampoos in a previous chapter.
7. Use a vinegar rinse.

Recipe I

3 Drops Lavender Essential oil

2 Drops Rosemary Essential oil

2 Drops West Indian Bay Essential oil

Recipe II

3 Drops Roman Chamomile Essential oil
2 Drops Thyme Essential oil
2 Drops Carrot Seed Essential oil

Recipe III

2 Drops Clary Sage Essential oil
2 Drops Cedarwood Essential oil
2 Drops Lavender Essential oil

Chapter 6 - Healthy Hair From the Inside

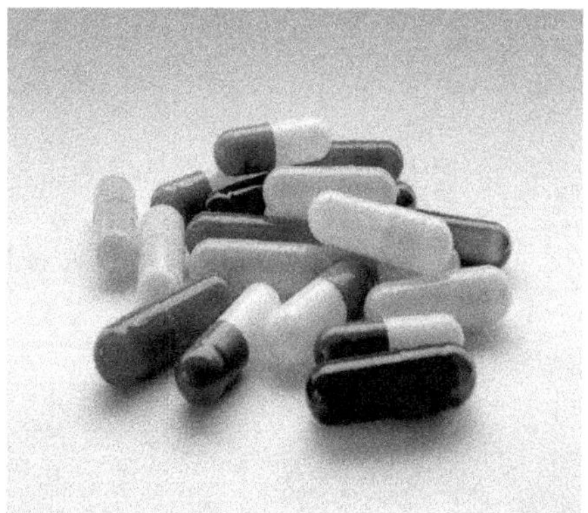

We've discussed how to tackle making your hair and scalp on the surface. In this chapter, I will go over some vitamins, minerals, and herbal supplements to help you get stronger and healthier hair from the inside.

Vitamins and minerals

Fish oils

This is high in Omega-3 fatty acids. It helps thicken the hair, and promote a healthy scalp.

Zinc

Zinc is instrumental to helping prevent the regression of hair follicles. It also helps to heal damaged and irritated follicles. Fun fact: Some people who suffer from alopecia have a zinc deficiency.

B-Complex, Biotin and B5

B-complex, in general, promotes healthy hair, but biotin and panatothenic acid (b5) help to speed healing of damaged hair from over styling.

Vitamin C

This helps slow the aging of the hair, preventing the hair from turning gray.

Iron

Adding iron-rich foods like Swiss chard, collard greens, egg yolks, beef, spinach, and beans, preferably navy and black beans.

Vitamin D

A deficiency of this vitamin can actually speed hair loss. On warm days, you can sit outside in the sun for about 15 minutes to absorb your daily dose. During the winter months, an herbal based Vitamin D is recommended with an intake of 10,000 units daily.

Herbals

Aloe Vera

This juice is packed with the vitamins and minerals to help promote healthy hair and hair growth.

Horsetail

This is a highly recommended herb for strengthening the hair and promoting hair growth. It's also good for strong nails, too.

Kelp

This herb has natural minerals that can help thicken and strengthen the hair. Combined with horsetail, it's a potent one-two punch for hair health and growth.

Conclusion

This is just to get you started. There are many more recipes to experiment with and try. There are online forums you can join which can help you make you own combinations and further tailor your hair health to your personal body's metabolism. I hope this book has helped answer many of your questions. Until next time...

www.ingramcontent.com/pod-product-compliance
Lightning Source LLC
Chambersburg PA
CBHW071242240726
48654CB00009B/1170